180
INSIDE OUT

Step-by-step guide
to turn your diet–and life–around!

Holly Meredith

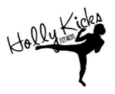

Important Legal Notice

Disclaimer

CONTENTS

Introduction

In my experience, there are three key components to making rapid and sustainable changes to your health. Nutrition, Exercise, and Mindset. One without the other might work for a short-term solution, but all three together is the key to making sustainable and life-long changes.

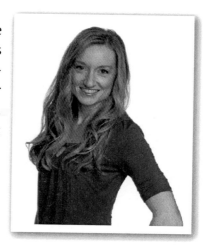

I have been a Health Coach and Fitness Instructor for over 7 years. I specialize in helping people achieve rapid and sustainable results - in a HEALTHY way.

Now you may be thinking... doesn't "rapid results" mean another "quick fix" that won't work? Not in this case. Rapid results AND sustainable results - it has to be both. Here's the deal, I find if my clients don't start seeing results right away, they give up. I mean our society is accustomed to instant gratification, right? So I'm going to give it to you. You'll likely see dramatic results in the very first week - and you'll break up with your old relationship with food. You'll be satiated and energized! THEN you'll learn how to tweak things to achieve sustainable, non-restrictive, lifelong habits.

We've been fed a myth for years that a healthy diet means eating low fat and high carbs. Imagine the food pyramid. Yet our USDA recommendations certainly haven't done anything to help our obesity rate - which interestingly enough has been on the rise since the food pyramid was adopted as our standard of eating. When I hear that this is STILL being taught in health classes today, and my children are being told that 65% of their diet should be from carbohydrates, and healthy fats like avocado and coconut oil will contribute to heart disease and weight gain - my head feels like it's about to explode!

It's time to break free of the fat-free craze! Non-fat, low-fat, it's a bunch of fat-free nonsense! And luckily the truth is now catching on.

Here's how a typical diet in our country goes...

- We eat too many carbs - stored as fat.

- We eat too much protein - stored as fat.

- We eat too few healthy fats - body stores it because it never gets enough.

- Think about it this way - we triple down on fat stores.

So, if you've followed the guidelines and loaded up on protein, fat free cereals, and skim milk, while also hitting the gym a few times a week, and your weight hasn't budged, and even likely increased - I'm here to flip everything you've been doing upside down and change your body. We're going to do a 180 - from the inside out.

The Plan

This plan pretty much goes against everything we've been told for years. But it also goes right along with what most of us know our bodies naturally want. When you learn scientifically WHY what we've been told is garbage, why we need to eat another way, why the way we've been told to eat isn't sustainable, and start learning to listen to our bodies - it's liberating.

I was pretty much at my ideal weight (give or take a couple lbs), was eating on point, working out a lot - and yet, I was bloated, my midsection no longer looked like it used to at that weight, my energy was crashing every day, naps became the norm, I wasn't FEELING my best, and I was frustrated.

What I used to do to look my best wasn't working anymore. I would stick closely to my food plan, no splurges, I even completed a 21 day cleanse - which did the trick, but wasn't a sustainable plan. A couple months later, I was stuck again. I didn't want to do another cleanse, and quite frankly, I shouldn't have to when I was on point with my nutrition and workouts...and yet my body wasn't responding.

Then my skin started breaking out. I didn't know what was going on with my skin, but I couldn't get it to stop. The last time I had skin problems was after years of pregnancies and breastfeeding and my hormones were all out of whack. Then I started on Shakeology and my skin cleared up within a month. This time was different though, and I was beyond frustrated.

I also wasn't sleeping well. It was hard to fall asleep and I was waking up several times a night - which I figured is why I needed a nap every day.

Probably, though, the biggest reason that I went on a mission to figure this problem out - I had long term clients who had been struggling. They previously had great success but then struggled to maintain that lifestyle. Starting again and falling off. Finding it hard to constantly eat well, and feeling like failures. Food temptation was a daily fight for them. They felt like they were doing something wrong. Like they didn't have enough willpower. And that is flat out demoralizing when you know something has worked before, but you just can't maintain it and feel like it's YOUR fault. I KNOW that's not how we're supposed to feel. For years I've blamed it on the food industry and the garbage in our food that's highly addictive, however, I'm no longer convinced that's the whole story.

I started experimenting on myself with a complete change to my diet. I also started practicing intermittent fasting. My results were so drastic that I started sharing the plan with my friends who were struggling. They also had wonderful results and broke through plateaus they had been stuck at for years, and even had blood work done to verify the internal changes to their thyroid levels and cholesterol. I then started coaching my clients through this way of eating, and over time, my approach has become clear:

- Eat low carbs, high fats, and a moderate amount of protein

- Practice Intermittent Fasting

- Achieve "fat adaption"

- Adjust your macros after 30 days to find the highest amount of carbs you can have while still achieving results

- Exercise

- Have a clear understanding about WHY you're following this plan so that you feel good about your choices and are empowered!

That's what you will learn in this book, with a step-by-step process.

Nutrition

WHAT IS A LOW CARB HIGH FAT DIET?

We've all heard of low-carb diets before such as Atkins or Paleo, but what makes the low-carb high-fat (LCHF) diet different is we're focusing on increasing our healthy fats as well, with moderate amounts of protein. The increase in fat and decrease in carbohydrates transitions your body from using glucose for energy, to fat for energy. When we use glucose for energy it's like a roller coaster for our blood sugar and it goes like this...

Eat —> feel an energy high —> crash —> crave more carbs —> eat —> energy —> crash —> crave more carbs —> repeat. Sound familiar?

When you eat a LCHF diet and your body becomes adapted at burning its own fat for fuel (fat adapted), it helps your blood sugar stabilize which causes sustained and even energy throughout the day. You'll no longer feel highs and lows and cravings throughout the day - instead, it's a constant even flow of energy! Check out the chart below:

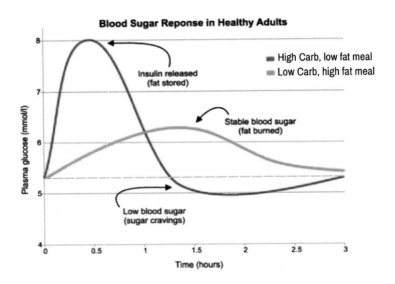

INTERMITTENT FASTING:

Intermittent Fasting is when you adjust your normal eating window to a smaller timeframe (ie: eating only between 10-6) instead of eating all day. This is becoming increasingly popular because it can help you lose weight without feeling hunger. You consume the same amount of calories but within a smaller time frame. A typical eating window may be from 10 AM - 6 PM, and the fast would be from 6 PM - 10 AM. When your body is without food for an extended period of time it will burn through its glycogen stores and be forced to burn it's own fat for energy. Plus, eating a LCHF diet gives your body fewer carbohydrates (glucose supply) to have to burn through. That's double downing on fat burning! Want to triple down? Add fasted workouts! Working out during your morning fast will cause your body to burn through the glycogen stores even quicker and access stored fat for energy. We'll get to more on workouts later though.

Here are some other good reasons to use IF. Along with weight loss, IF has been shown to decrease diabetes, heart disease, increase energy, and also lead to a better night's sleep. In fact, this way of eating was practiced by our ancestors because they didn't have endless amounts of food around like we do now.

In my opinion, the most practical and awesome thing about IF is no longer having your life revolve around food. I always felt like I was on a food marathon throughout the day. Most diet plans have you eating 5-6 times per day, all day, and a LOT of food. If I got home late in the morning after teaching classes I knew there was no way I was going to have time to eat all the food I was allotted for the day. And even though I was eating every 1-2 hours, I would get HUNGRY because the low-fat/non-fat food wasn't satiating. I would always pack snacks with me everywhere I went. I've never thought so much about food than when I was "on plan" and thought I was eating right.

When I said we are going to do a 180 from everything we've been doing - I really meant it! I know - we've been told we need to eat a lot of small meals throughout the day to lose weight! We do NOT need to be eating all the time. And that's where hormone health comes into play with IF.

We all have hunger hormones - ghrelin and leptin. Ghrelin is the hormone that tells us when we're hungry and leptin is the hormone that gives us the feeling of being full. Both are important. There's a reason we have hormones in our bodies, and to have proper levels we need to let our bodies go through the natural process of actually getting hungry. We are supposed to let our bodies feel hungry, then feel satisfied, and then get hungry again. If you skip that process and constantly eat - insulin, ghrelin, and leptin don't do their jobs and we don't get the hormone balance we need - which then causes weight gain. In short, we cannot constantly feed our face!

At first, many people are afraid they won't be able to eat only within an 8-hour window. Think back though...if you're like most of my clients, skipping breakfast used to be the norm. Yet, we've been told "breakfast is the most important meal of the day!" and so I've hounded many clients to EAT BREAKFAST! I didn't naturally like eating breakfast either. I trained my body to eat breakfast and you probably did too. We can also train our bodies to wait, and eat breakfast later.

As you get started with IF, consider taking it slow. You might start with LCHF and then add IF later. It is much easier to do IF once your body is fat adapted and no longer searching for carbs. Some people start with everything on day one, some don't. This is an individual preference. Some people may find transitioning to IF extremely challenging - your body will adapt. So, if you wake up starving and have no idea how you're going to ever get to an 8-hour eating window...take it slow and consider the following:

Week 1: Eating within a 12-hour window

Week 2: Eating within a 10-hour window

Week 3: and beyond: Eating within an 8-hour window

We all live busy lives and our schedules change. Don't beat yourself up if your eating window is longer on one day than another. We do the best we can with the schedules we have.

KETOSIS/NUTRITIONAL KETOSIS:

Ketosis is the metabolic state in which the body is using fat for energy. It's a normal metabolic process that happens when there is a lack of carbohydrates from food, and therefore the body turns to burning it's own fat for energy. When the body metabolizes fat, ketones are created and the ketone molecules are used for energy.

The primary focus of this plan is not Ketosis. HOWEVER, eating low carb high fat and practicing intermittent fasting CAN put you into Nutritional Ketosis. What is the difference? The word "Nutritional". Basically, nutritional ketosis is a state of health where the body is fed a wide array of nutrients AND efficiently burning fat as its primary fuel source rather than glucose. If the goal is ONLY to get into ketosis, many people fall into the trap of cutting out vital nutrients to see high levels of ketones in their body (I'll get to more on that later). In this picture, I used a test to measure the amounts of ketones in my body - and you can see that my body had a moderate amount of ketones. What I'm showing you is that I do indeed have ketones even after having Shakeology! Many people think you cannot have Shakeology (even though it's only 11-14 g net carbs per serving) and stay in ketosis. Yeah...you can. In fact, it's the healthiest most nutrient dense form of carbo-hydrates you can put into your body packed with over 70 superfoods! Proof - you can eat healthy, nutrient dense foods and STILL be fat adapted.

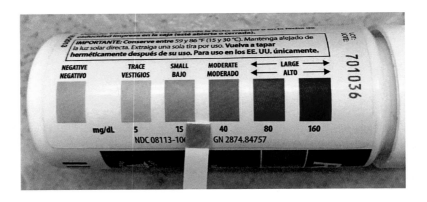

How do you know if you're in Ketosis?

If you're seeing weight-loss, full of energy, and feeling satiated - congratulations - you're likely in ketosis! I compare the feeling to adrenaline. I feel full of energy, my body is in an excited-awake state, I find myself buzzing around the house, and feel like I can get a thousand things done at once! If you're interested in testing to be sure, see the FAQ's for more information about test strips.

In the beginning, there are usually side effects as your body becomes fat adapted. It can last from a couple of days to a few weeks. Expect to feel short-term fatigue, short-term decreased exercise performance, possibly flu-like symptoms referred to as the "keto-flu", and digestive issues. For most people it takes a few days, then they get their energy rush and know they're in ketosis. It took five days for my husband, 6 days for me. I woke up on day six and had more energy than I've ever had in my life!

You can help combat the initial side effects by drinking plenty of water, and supplementing with magnesium usually helps alleviate constipation as your body adjusts.

I HIGHLY suggest sticking closely to plan and powering through the initial side effects to get into nutritional ketosis as quickly as possible. If you waffle on plan it will just drag the process out longer.

SHAKEOLOGY

I recommend Shakeology for the majority of daily carbs. I would say the MOST important thing I do for my health is drink Shakeology every day. In fact, I don't even feel comfortable coaching people through the way I'm eating without it. Why? Because I'm just not interested in working with people whose sole goal is to lose weight, even at the expense of their health. Cutting out something like Shakeology to achieve lower carbs makes ZERO sense to me.

When you're limiting your carbohydrate intake it's very important to make sure you get the most bang for your buck, or in this case, carb. I have not found a better source for such condensed nutrition (micronutrients) in only 11-14 grams of net carbs than Shakeology. Micronutrients, as opposed to macronutrients (protein, carbohydrates and fat), are vitamins and minerals which are required in small quantities for normal metabolism, growth and physical well-being. This is super important! If you're fed enough calories AND enough micronutrients (it has to be both) your body doesn't feel like it's in an emergency and it will let go of fat! So, if you skip your Shakeology to save on carbs, your body is likely to hold onto fat because it's not getting enough nutrients. Your body needs the consistency so it will release what it doesn't need. Make sense? You've got to have BOTH; calories AND micronutrients. And that's why I'm not only at my leanest - but why I also FEEL better than ever. I can't stress this enough - be on a quest for a healthy weight AND a healthy body!

Isn't fat bad?

Not healthy fats! The ever popular low fat-high carb diet that we've been told is healthy, is actually the complete opposite of what we need to prevent disease and OPTIMIZE our health. Healthy fat doesn't make you fat or raise your bad cholesterol levels - sugar does. Even if you're thinking that you don't eat much sugar, remember, sugar comes in many forms besides just sugary foods - it's also in almost every processed food, milk, grain products, excess fruit, and even excess protein. You see, dietary cholesterol has nothing to do with blood cholesterol, so avoiding healthy fats isn't helping anyone's cholesterol levels. Cardiologist, Steven Nissan, says "About 85 percent of the cholesterol in the circulation is manufactured by the body in the liver, it isn't coming directly from the cholesterol that you eat."

Instead, try cutting out the carbs and see what happens! Thank goodness it's finally being acknowledged that low-fat isn't the way to go - because we've been needlessly avoiding things like eggs and avocado - and our health is none the better for it!

WHY DOES THE GOVERNMENT SAY THAT FAT IS BAD?

Policy makers have told us to avoid eggs and healthy fats because cholesterol and fat are bad. Luckily, that terrible advice is continually being proved wrong and the truth is slowly becoming mainstream.

In the 1970's, it was hypothesized by Dr. Ancel Keys that dietary saturated fat caused heart disease and should be avoided. He conducted a study in countries where people's diets were higher in saturated fats and where they also had a higher rate of heart disease. Here's the kicker - Dr. Keys ONLY searched for populations and evidence that supported his hypothesis! And through those findings, he concluded that saturated fat causes heart disease. Shockingly enough, that was the study that initiated the low-fat dietary guidelines.

I think you'll agree, sloppy science should no longer guide the American nutrition policy. We have cut down on meat and eggs (fat and protein) while we increased grains, pasta, rice, starchy vegetables (carbohydrates) and watched the obesity rates rise right along with it. It's actually a very scary domino effect. We've been told to eat more carbohydrates than any other food group, yet carbohydrates cause blood glucose to rise the most and the most quickly. When we eat too much glucose and our cells already have filled glycogen stores, the excess glucose is stored as fat. How do you stop this process? Stop the insulin spikes caused by eating excess carbohydrates - and eat more healthy fats causing our bodies to become fat burning machines!

The good news is - we don't have to wait for new dietary guidelines to change our own diets. It's a free country! We can be empowered with our own knowledge and demolish the "fat makes you fat" myth.

How is this different than other diets?

Many people have heard of "low carb" diets such as Keto, Paleo, and Atkins. In my opinion, those are missing some very key components.

Dr. Atkins did a great job of bringing the spotlight to the low carb diet, but unfortunately, he stopped there - and didn't also focus on increasing healthy fats. When cutting down on carbohydrates it's imperative to also increase the healthy fats. When your body is fed enough healthy fats, it becomes satiated and no longer craving carbs.

The Paleo diet has been great for bringing awareness to the health benefits of being grain-free. However, much of the focus tends to be on high amounts of protein. Our bodies, our muscles, just do not need that much protein. The average American eats much more protein than their body can utilize.

In the Keto diet, the primary goal is to be in ketosis to burn fat for fuel. Excellent - except many keto dieters cut out nutritious carbs (including all fruits, and even many veggies) for the purpose of staying ultra low carb. Their thinking is that if their carbs are super low, then they'll reach high levels of ketones in their body and therefore burn more fat. Your body does NOT need to have high levels of ketones to be in a fat burning state. Quite frankly, that's just flat out not healthy behavior. We need a variety of nutrient dense foods for our bodies to have all our vitamins, minerals, antioxidants, etc! Without it, you will do more harm than good to your organs and your health.

Our focus is on optimal health with fat adaption - which will produce results far more reaching than just weight loss. So, this is not Keto, Paleo, Atkins, or anything else. This is a healthy, balanced, and sustainable approach. I built this plan with my values, with what I've found works, and with what I will stand behind.

- I'm a mom

- I'm here to set an example

- I'm about health

- I'm about results

- But I'm not here to get you skinny at the expense of your health.

How much protein do we really need?

On the left is me before starting this plan. On the right is me after 8 weeks of following this plan. I've leaned out and gained muscle. And my diet is not heavy on protein. I know, we all think we need so much protein - to build muscle and stay satiated...it's not true. The average American eats way more protein than they need - and when your body can't utilize the amount you eat at that time, it can be turned into glucose just like if you were eating more carbs - a process called gluconeogenesis.

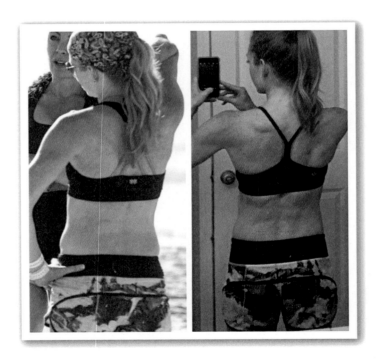

Reducing carbs, upping healthy fats, and *gasp* reducing protein - all are key. You guys, our society isn't protein deficient, we're nutrient deficient.

WHAT IS CONSIDERED "LOW CARBOHYDRATES"?

A LCHF diet means you're limiting your carbohydrates to approximately 20% of your daily calories. We begin the plan with lower carbs to test insulin sensitivity (sometimes around 10%) then INCREASE once your body is fat adapted (approx 2-3 weeks). This will vary based on individual goals and insulin resistance (how easily your body will release weight).

After calculating protein and carbs, healthy fats will make up the rest approximately 50% or more of your daily calories.

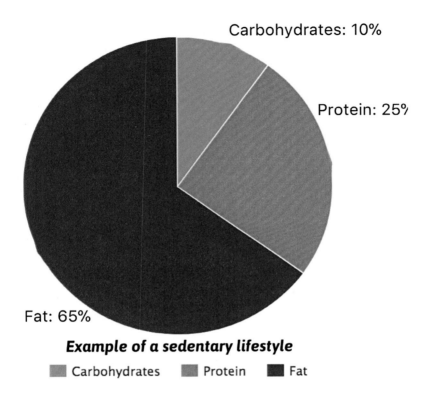

Example of a sedentary lifestyle

Carbohydrates   Protein   Fat

HOW DO I GET STARTED?

Everyone begins with the same 7 Day Plan. You can make some alterations, ie: swap out one green veggie for another, or use another meat besides bacon, etc. The calories on this plan are close enough to the caloric range for most people - so everyone begins here. The point of the 7 Day Plan is to test your insulin sensitivity. It's meant to transition your body to using fat for fuel, so it's important to follow it closely to get your body fat adapted as soon as possible. If you follow the plan loosely it will take longer to understand the process, longer for fat adaption to occur, which can lead both to confusion, frustration, and ultimately feeling defeated. That's why I specialize in RAPID results. Not because I want to promote a "quick fix", but because the quicker people see results, the more motivated people become - the more knowledge and experience people have, the more empowered they feel. So, I want you to get right to it, experience it, see results, learn about your body, and be motivated to continue!

See Appendix for the 7 Day Plan.

WHAT DO I DO AFTER DAY 7?

After day 7, use the chart in Appendix 1 to calculate your macros. Macros = broad categories of food, like protein, carbs, fat. You can start eating different foods beyond the 7 day plan, but make sure they fit within your macros.

I highly suggest downloading an app to track everything you eat for this next part as you get started. (See the FAQ's for app suggestions) This should not be a forever thing, but it will help you in the beginning to understand the macros in the 7-day plan which will help you start to get an understanding of which foods are your source of carbs, protein, and fats. Some foods might surprise you as to what they do to your macros and you'll make adjustments. That might sound overwhelming at first - but once you start tracking, all of a sudden you "get" it. Remember - knowledge is power - and understanding your body is probably the most important power you can have. Once you understand it, quit tracking and just pay attention to your body and how you feel!

TIP:

Sometimes before I decide what I'm going to eat I will enter the food into my app to see what the different options do to my macros. Then I choose based on which one fulfills my needs for the day.

The next few weeks are going to solidify becoming fat adapted. This process can take anywhere from 1-3 weeks for most people, so it's important to stick closely to your macros during this first month.

CARB REFEEDS/CARB-UPS:
WHY DO WE NEED THEM?

The insulin spike from high glycemic foods (carbs) resets ghrelin and leptin hormones and aids in the production of T4 (thyroid hormone) as well as converting T4 to T3 (useable energy from T4). We don't want our bodies to think carbs are so scarce that they start converting muscles to glucose through glucogenesis. When people stay LCHF for long periods of time and never do refeeds they tend to immediately gain weight when they have carbs. We need to make sure our bodies don't forget how to metabolize carbs, so to speak. Once your body is fat adapted it handles the small cycles of carbs much more easily - in fact when you do a refeed you will likely find that your body will metabolize the carbs faster than ever and you'll wake up even leaner. This is a very important part of making this a lifestyle - and a plan that doesn't stop working after long periods of time. Carbs are not the enemy, we just don't need a constant high dose of them wreaking havoc on our bodies.

WHEN TO DO THEM:

Once you're fat adapted AND feeling like you need carbs (usually after 2-3 weeks) then start carb refeeds.

HOW TO DO THEM:

It really depends on your relationship with food.

If having carbs tends to set you off on a downward spiral to eating everything in sight, then you probably want to plan them and be very mindful.

Example: One high carb meal every Sunday night. Back to plan Monday morning.

If being too strict freaks you out and you tend to rebel, then do carbs every now and then without planning and make them your way of not feeling restricted.

Example: Out to dinner at a Mexican restaurant and you have the tortilla with your meal, two days later you have some sweet potatoes at lunch, over the weekend you have dessert out with friends.

WHAT TO EAT:

Ideally, it would be foods like sweet potatoes, fruit, carrots - no grains. Having said that, I typically have a high carb meal on Sunday night including ice cream.

HOW OFTEN:

Generally once every 7-10 days, lasting one evening. Some women need them every 4 days.

How often really depends on the level of body fat left to lose, metabolism, goals, etc. Talk to me so we can make an individual plan!

TIP:

In my experience, after I eat extra carbs I tend to start craving them again the next day. To combat that, make sure you're having extra fats the next morning - also just knowing the cravings might happen will help you move through them instead of thinking that something has gone wrong. It will pass.

Important Reminder:

We are here to create a LIFESTYLE that actually works to keep our bodies running at their best with the best energy source. I highly recommend making sure your body is fat adapted, then cycling in carbs regularly. And above all - listen to your body.

AFTER 30 DAYS:

> You've completed the initial 7-day plan ✓
> You've started tracking your macros ✓
> You've been around 50 g of daily carbs ✓
> You've started doing regular carb refeeds ✓

Now what?

It's time to start increasing your daily carbohydrate intake. The goal is to find the sweet spot where you can have the highest amount of carbs, while still seeing results.

Start by increasing just 5 grams of extra carbohydrates per day for one week, then do a refeed. The following week you'll add an extra 5 grams, then do a refeed. The following week you'll add an extra 5 grams, and so on.

Here is an example of what month two might look like:

Week 1: Increase to 55 grams of total carbohydrates, no change

Week 2: Increase to 60 grams of total carbohydrates, no change

Week 3: Increase to 65 grams of total carbohydrates with wild rice added, noticeable change (bloating, acid reflux, no energy)

Week 4: 65 grams of total carbohydrates (without wild rice), minimal change

So, in this example, this person knows their sweet spot is between 60-65 grams of carbohydrates, but possibly not from grains. Keep experimenting.

Make it a goal to experiment on yourself. For example; try adding a serving of fruit, then see how your body feels. Maybe you can eat a serving of fruit once a day, maybe that makes you bloated, but you can eat it a few times per week - what you do one day does not need to be the same as the next day. However, when changing your overall macros try and give it about 5-7 days to really see how you're body is going to respond.

After you find your sweet spot and beyond:

The MOST import-ant thing to remem-ber is you're doing this for your health AND your life. If you feel like having something spe-cific to eat, maybe you should go ahead and have it (after your body is fat adapted). If you feel like you could use extra carbs one day - have a sweet potato. If 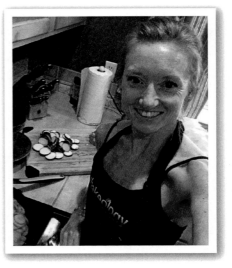 you receive chocolates, have them. Then get back to your plan because this is your PLAN, not a diet. Your body wants to be at a healthy weight, so once you're using fat for fuel your body should burn the extra splurges easily.

If not, figure out what would work better for YOU next time. THERE IS NO ONE PLAN FOR EVERYBODY. Be your own experiment - and eventually, you'll break FREE from counting and tracking altogether.

Workouts

Here's the deal - stress and weight gain go hand in hand. Chronic stress has been called the "silent killer" as it's a major contributing factor to the six leading causes of death in the US. It wreaks so much havoc on our health - and yet the best and most natural stress reliever is SIMPLE. I didn't say easy, I said simple. Exercise! Exercise lowers levels of anxiety, depression, and stress. That's even true for those who are stressed out by the idea of exercise. It's literally the most natural stress reliever out there!

Not only that, but movement creates energy! We all want more energy, we want to feel vibrant, right? Then we've got to get up and MOVE our bodies.

OK, hopefully, I've convinced you now.

You do not need to stop exercising as you get started with this plan. However, during the first couple of weeks eating LCHF, you might feel very sluggish during your workouts. My legs felt heavy and they would burn just going up 2 flights of stairs! Don't worry - it gets better. In fact, after a few weeks, you should start to notice that you are able to lift heavier and workout with more endurance than you had before.

What kind of workouts you do depends very much on your fitness level, health, injuries, etc. Please contact me for a customized plan. In general, make sure you're getting at least 30 minutes of exercise at least three times per week. Yeah, it doesn't have to be as much as many people think.

Here are some ideas…

Just beginning?

Get out and walk!

Start a Couch to 5 K walk/run program (you can find those free online).

Start the PiYo home workout program (excellent low-impact workout).

Already active?

Get out and run!

Do a home workout program from start to finish (you'll feel very accomplished checking off each day).

Here is the breakdown I recommend:

- HIIT (High Intensity Interval Training) workouts 2-3 times per week - this is all out, barely able to catch your breath, 100% effort workouts for about 25-30 minutes per session. The idea is to get so anaerobic that your body must work for hours afterward to come back to its natural resting state. We call that "afterburn". The type of exercise depends on your fitness level and what puts you into that anaerobic zone - this might be fast walking for some people, sprinting or squat jumps for others.

- Strength workouts 2-3 times per week. Strength workouts can be anything from lifting weights to yoga, pilates, swimming, bodyweight exercises - so many options.

- Make sure to take a rest day.

You might remember me mentioning "fasted workouts" in the Intermittent Fasting section. This is when you do your workout outside of your eating window. Think of it as triple downing on your fat burning. Here's what I mean... First, you started restricting your carbs (glucose) so your body has less of it to use. Second, you started practicing IF so your body runs out of glycogen stores and is forced to burn its own fat stores for energy. Third, you add a workout during your fast so your body must access even more fat stores for energy - faster fat burning for you!

Many people worry they will be fatigued and light-headed if they don't eat before they workout. That sensation happens when your body is looking for glucose for energy. Once your body is fat adapted and not looking for glucose you should no longer feel that sensation. Eventually, you'll be able to workout during your fast and have more energy than ever before.

Whether you do fasted workouts or not, you will

reap rewards. Some days you might be able to do fasted workouts, some days your schedule might now allow for it. Don't let your eating window dictate whether or not you workout. It's too important to skip!

Fitness is about so much more than exercise. It's a catalyst for positive changes, and it affects every aspect of your life.

Mindset

"The secret of change is to focus all of your energy, not on fighting the old, but on building the new."

—Dan Millman,
Way of the Peaceful Warrior

I believe having a healthy mindset is the third pillar of success when it comes to health.

So, let's start by discussing the mindset of the "D" word. Diet.

Someone asked why I would be dieting when I don't need to lose weight. That is sort of the way our society thinks, right? That eating healthy, in proper portions, proper balance, and in a way that makes you feel good... that's a diet. Ok. Then I'm on a diet. Along with the healthiest people I've known for years who use their diet to prevent things like cancer, autoimmune diseases, digestion issues, and a world of other illnesses that send so many to the doctor annually. The problem is most people think of a diet as a way to lose weight. Losing weight is actually a side effect of all the wonderful things your body will do when it's fed properly. It's about finally figuring out how your body works. It's about realizing why you've been craving junk all the time. It's eating in a way that those feelings of either obsessing over food or depriving yourself of food go away. It's being empowered to know that just because our society says something is "normal" doesn't make it so (ie; Doritos, Twinkies, energy drinks, any junk food that people accept as the norm). Just because companies want to make money and put food in our faces doesn't mean that's normal eating and if you eat differently you're weird. For real, someone said "it's a little extreme to NEVER eat Doritos" Huh?!! Why? Because the Doritos company exists I need to eat it? I think that's really weird, and yet that's how many people feel. And it's with that mentality that someone asked me why I would "diet". My passion is helping people who have had enough of being bloated (sometimes to the point of their skin hurting), decrease sex drive, diarrhea or constipation, bad skin, no energy, terrible periods, and so on - through changing their DIET. In fact, I would say, be PROUD of your diet! It's your choice after all, and you're free to change your mind at any time.

> *"She is clothed in Strength and Dignity"*
>
> —*Proverbs 31-25*

When we complain about how we have to eat, exercise, or the schedule we have to keep to get the results we want

- that's not helpful, and it's certainly not dignified. I truly believe that when we feel acceptance and gratitude for our choices, we release resentment and our bodies respond more quickly.

> "You've gotten to where you are right now by doing whatever it is you're doing. So, if you're less than impressed with your current situation, you clearly need to change things up."
>
> —Jen Sincero

Set a new STANDARD for yourself. People make goals all the time without actually achieving them. But you know what we always achieve? We achieve our standards. If you look at an athlete, their standard is eating a certain way, having a certain amount of endurance or strength, and they are unwavering in what it takes to maintain that standard. Look at the income standards people set for themselves. They will work extremely hard to make sure they reach certain numbers at the end of the month when it's their standard of living on the line. This also goes to small stuff like the standard of clothing you buy, how green you keep your grass, and so on. Whatever standards you have adopted for yourself you meet. For me, when there are no food options that meet my standard, I won't eat. I will wait until I can get something that meets my standards. If someone is following a plan just to meet a weight loss goal, they will probably throw in the towel and eat what's available because eating properly is not their standard, they merely have a goal and the time it takes to achieve that goal can change. I have standards that I won't compromise. So, really give some thought to what your standard for your health is.

Remember, you control your body, it does not control you.

I think in our society we have become resigned to the idea that we can't control ourselves; our cravings, our motivation level, our habits, or even the way our body moves. But we do have control. We were born with an innate ability to use our brain to signal our body, not just let our bodies or life happen to us. We can re-train our patterns, our habits, our bodies, we even have the ability to heal ourselves...we just have to decide to take that first step and start BELIEVING in ourselves. Maybe it's time to ask yourself when you started believing whatever story has been holding you back. What if you told yourself a new story... "I used to be a carb junkie, but now that's no longer who I am".

In my years of teaching group exercise, there's one thing I know - it's much more about your mindset than your body. We can talk ourselves out of working hard, decide we can only lift a certain amount, only do a certain amount of reps, tell ourselves that we need a break, or talk ourselves out of exercising at all. What if it was life or death though... COULD you do more? The answer is almost always, yes. Our minds give up well before our bodies do. It's actually a battle of the mind! Keep telling yourself you CAN and your body will follow. Next time you workout try repeating this mantra: "I can, I will, I am!" Because you CAN do it, so you WILL do it, and then you'll find you ARE doing it. Before you know it - you'll be done. Change your perspective and you'll change your life.

As you continue through this process, remember the power of your own words. If you come at this with the attitude of "Fine, I'll try this, but this is my last chance", or "let's see if this can actually work, because nothing else has", guess what? That's expecting failure and you're going to get back the energy you put out - failure. I can pretty much tell who's going to fail before they even start. It's that negativity, that complaining, that looking for reasons to give up before they even start - it's a self-fulfilling prophecy and they will prove themselves right.

There will be days when your macros are off. Maybe a few days at a time, maybe a whole vacation. So, what do you do? Most people say things like "I failed", "I fell off the wagon", "I got way off track". Stop looking at this as "off track" or "on track". It's one track, and it's going to be like a winding road. I can pretty much guarantee that! So, when things do go awry, instead of saying "I fell off the wagon", how about saying "I've had too many carbs lately to continue seeing results". One makes you feel like a failure, one makes you feel in control. And you ARE in control. Like I said before - YOU control your body, it does NOT control you.

> *"To reach up for the new, you must let go of the old. What lies behind you is not nearly as important as what lies in front of you. Everything you've been through was preparation for where you are right now."*
>
> —Joel Osteen

When you do the things that make you feel healthy, you enjoy being healthy. It's not about depriving yourself, it's like IGNITING yourself. Choose to do the things that give you more energy! Remember - you don't HAVE to do these things, you are CHOOSING to. You are never stuck, you have the freedom to do something different at any time.

I'm telling you - once you feel this vitality in your body, find a new level of your fitness, and set a new standard for yourself - that's when you'll never go back.

I am excited to share this gift with you. It has helped me in so many ways, I truly cannot wait for you to see and feel all the benefits of your own transformation. Please reach out to me personally. I'm here to help, and I'd love to help you find you own personal path through Nutrition, Exercise, and Mindset.

APPENDIX

7 Day Meal Plan

Monday	Tuesday	Wednesday	Thursday	Friday	Saturday	Sunday
2 organic pastured eggs 2 Tsp avocado oil 2 Tsp grass fed butter 1 cup spinach 1 slice cheddar cheese 1/4 avocado	2 organic pastured eggs 2 oz smoked salmon 2 TBS cream cheese 1/4 avocado	2 organic pastured eggs 1 TBS grass fed butter 3 slices organic pastured bacon 1/4 avocado	2 organic pastured eggs 2 Tsp avocado oil 2 Tsp grass fed butter 1 cup spinach 1 slice cheddar cheese 1/4 avocado	2 organic pastured eggs 2 oz smoked salmon 2 TBS cream cheese 1/4 avocado	2 organic pastured eggs 2 Tsp avocado oil 2 Tsp grass fed butter 1 cup spinach 1 slice cheddar cheese 1/4 avocado	2 organic pastured eggs 1 TBS grass fed butter 3 slices organic pastured bacon 1/4 avocado
		1 Scoop Shakeology 8 oz Unsweetened Coconut milk 2 Tsp coconut oil 1 TBS peanut butter				
6 oz organic grass fed steak 1 TBS organic grass fed butter 1/2 cup raw or roasted broccoli 1/2 cup raw or roasted zuchinni 1/2 cup raw or roasted cauliflower	2 cups romaine lettuce 3 oz organic free range chicken 1/4 cup bleu or feta cheese 1 hardboiled egg 1/2 cup cucumber 1/2 chopped tomato 1/4 avocado 2 Tbs organic cream based dressing (ie: bleu cheese, ranch)	6 oz grilled wild caught salmon 2 TBS organic grass fed butter 1.5 cups raw or steamed broccoli 1 oz organic sharp cheddar cheese	6 oz organic free range chicken breast 2 Tbs organic grass fed butter 12 raw or roasted asparagus spears	6 oz organic grass fed steak 1 TBS organic grass fed butter 1/2 cup raw or roasted broccoli 1/2 cup raw or roasted zuchinni 1/2 cup raw or roasted cauliflower	2 cups romaine lettuce 3 oz organic free range chicken breast 1/4 cup bleu or feta cheese 1 hardboiled egg 1/2 cup cucumber 1/2 chopped tomato 1/4 avocado 2 Tbs organic cream based dressing (ie: bleu cheese, ranch)	6 oz grilled wild caught salmon 2 TBS organic grass fed butter 1.5 cups raw or steamed broccoli 1 oz organic sharp cheddar cheese
Calories: 1391 Fat:104 g Carbs: 39 g Protein: 78 g	Calories: 1383 Fat: 96 g Carbs: 41 g Protein: 90 g	Calories: 1442 Fat: 105 g Carbs: 42 g Protein: 90 g	Calories: 1426 Fat: 100 g Carbs: 39 g Protein: 98 g	Calories: 1400 Fat: 102 g Carbs: 41 g Protein: 86 g	Calories: 1384 Fat: 100 g Carbs: 34 g Protein: 84 g	Calories: 1442 Fat: 105 g Carbs: 42 g Protein: 90 g

CALCULATING CALORIES & MACROS
STEP 1 - CALCULATE TOTAL DAILY CALORIES:

Multiply your target weight by 10-11 for a sedentary lifestyle.

Multiply your target weight by 12-13 for a moderately active lifestyle.

Multiply your target weight by 14-15 for an active lifestyle.

STEP 2 - CALCULATE PROTEIN:

Choose protein percentage from the chart.

Multiply daily calories by protein percentage

Example: Daily calories 1800 x .25 (25% protein) = 450 calories

Divide protein calories by 4 to get daily grams of protein (because there are 4 calories per gram of protein)

Example: 450/4 = 112.5 grams of protein per day

STEP 3 - CALCULATE CARBOHYDRATES:

Multiply daily calories by .20 (20% carbs)

Example: Daily calories 1800 x .20 = 360

Divide carbohydrate calories by 4 to get daily grams of carbs (because there are 4 calories per gram of carbs)

Example: 360/4 = 90 grams of carbs per day

STEP 4 - CALCULATE FATS:

All remaining calories go to fat.

Example: Daily calories 1800, subtract 450 calories from protein, subtract 360 calories from carbohydrates, leaving 990 calories from fat.

Divide fat calories by 9 to get daily grams of fat (because there are 9 calories per gram of fat)

Example: 990/9 = 110 grams of fats per day

These calculations will put you at 20% carbs, you can start there if you'd like because 20% carbs is certainly considered low-carb, but the recommended number of carbs to become fat adapted is 50 grams or less of total carbs. That means, for most people, you will be BELOW 20% of your calories in carbs to start. So, when you calculate you'll need to drop your carbs a little lower than 20% to be at 50 g or lower. If that is your goal, then decrease your carbs - increase your fat - and leave the protein alone (no more than 30%). That is why I recommend you use a customizable tracking app. Please refer to the charts below to figure the appropriate amount of carbs based on your lifestyle.

Carbohydrate Guide

ACTIVITY LEVEL	DAILY GRAMS	PERCENTAGE % OF TOTAL CALORIES
Sedentary	<20	10-15
Active Lifestyle	20-50	15-20
Endurance Athlete	50-100	20-25

Protein Guide

ACTIVITY LEVEL	PERCENTAGE % OF TOTAL CALORIES
Sedentary	15
Active Lifestyle	20
Weight Lifter	25

Fat Guide

FAT WILL MAKE UP THE REST OF THE DAILY CALORIES
50%-80%

Using me as an example:

Protein: 135 g (29%)
Carbs: 51 g (11%)
Fat: 124 g (60%)

You can see that if I had my carbs at 20% I would be much higher than 50 g.

*You can adjust and customize your macros in the MyNetDiary Pro version or My FitnessPal and it will change the grams/percentages for you.

FOOD SOURCES

Following the initial 7 day plan and tracking in an app will give you a really good baseline for what food sources are appropriate for your macros.

Protein: Look for organic pastured eggs, grass-fed organic meat, and wild caught fish. While a little bit of bacon here and there is fine, it shouldn't be the norm. You will do much better by avoiding processed meats, including lunch meat. I'm not a vegetarian, so I'm not the best resource for vegetarian protein sources, but if you consume tofu I would suggest organic and fermented and only consume it occasionally.

Carbohydrates: The majority of your carbs will come from your Shakeology. Beyond that, I suggest nut butter, coconut milk, and green leafy vegetables. For vegetables, think of veggies that grow above ground. The root vegetables (like carrots and sweet potatoes) are higher in carbs. When adding fruit, look for the most nutritious and lowest in carbs (blueberries, raspberries, blackberries).

Fats: This is the fun part - many of the things you thought were off-limits, you can have! Avocados, egg yolks, coconut oil, olive oil, grass-fed butter, ghee, hard cheese, heavy cream. Remember - while we are eating a high-fat diet, this means HEALTHY fats.

FAQ's

WHAT APP DO YOU RECOMMEND FOR TRACKING MACROS?

My favorite app is MyNetDiary Pro, $3.99. It allows you to customize your calories and macros, as opposed to apps that give you a default based on simplistic stats like height and weight. You can slide the carbs down to 50g and it will automatically increase the protein and fats. Then you can slide the protein down and it will automatically increase the fats. Other great apps: My Fitness Pal, Carb Manager. I'm sure there are many others as well.

WHAT IS INSULIN SENSITIVITY/RESISTANCE?

People with insulin resistance are unable to pull glucose into the cells, which means that excess glucose builds up in the blood causing higher than normal blood sugar levels. With nowhere else to go, the body turns this extra energy into fat and stores it for later.

WILL EXTRA VEGGIES PUT ME OUT OF NUTRITIONAL KETOSIS?

Green veggies are not going to take you out of fat burning. If green veggies put you over your carbs, don't worry about it. However, in the beginning if you're consistently over 50 g carbs, I would look at the other carbs in your diet and consider cutting them out. For example, many people add nuts or a post workout drink, but then cut back on veggies to achieve 50 g. I would reduce the other carbs before reducing veggies. If it's mostly veggies making up your carbs then don't worry about them putting you over. No one is going to gain weight from eating veggies. The goal is health, not meeting certain numbers.

Is THERE A RIGHT OR WRONG TIME TO EAT YOUR MACROS?

It's best to eat more fats earlier in the day when your body is in its highest fat burning state. Save the carbs for later in the day, which will also help you sleep better.

Do I HAVE TO PRACTICE INTERMITTENT FASTING FOR THIS PLAN TO WORK?

Not at all. It will help you achieve fat adaption faster, but if you want to start with either LCHF or IF, then I would choose LCHF first. Once your body is fat adapted you'll find it's easier to add IF than when your body is looking for glucose for energy.

What is BulletProof coffee?

It's typically coffee with butter and medium-chain triglycerides from coconut oil added. Basically, adding healthy fats to your coffee. Here's how I personally make it:

12 oz organic coffee
1 tsp Madagascar Vanilla Ghee
2 tsp Brain Octane MCT oil
3 TBS heavy cream
Blend - and you have a delicious healthy drink!

Does BulletProof coffee break your fast?

Some people say as long as you consume less than 50 calories it's OK. Some people say since BP coffee is only healthy fats which won't cause an insulin response it's OK. My opinion is that your body will use what's in your stomach first. So, really anything will halt fat burning and therefore BP coffee will break your fast. Having said that, if I'm having a day when I feel particularly hungry in the morning I might have my BP coffee early. Especially on the days when I've had carbs the night before and my body feels off. It can be an effective way of getting extra fats early in the day and combatting the carb cravings after a re-feed.

WHEN I BURN CALORIES DURING EXERCISE, DOES THAT MEAN I CAN EAT THAT MANY MORE CALORIES DURING THE DAY?

It really doesn't work that way. If it did, then everyone who exercises would basically be able to eat an entire extra meal per day. Your workouts help build strong muscles, cardiovascular health, balance, endurance, spinal alignment, skeletal support, mental wellness, and so much more. Your food is for nourishment. I would say, let your food be your food, and your exercise be your exercise.

IF I'M ALREADY LEAN, SHOULD I STILL ADD FASTED WORKOUTS?

Even if you're already lean you will reap the rewards of fasted workouts. Remember, each facet of this plan is about more than weight loss, it's about creating optimal health and energy! So, if you're worried about losing too much weight, let's take a super ripped 150 lb man with 8% body fat. Even at 8% body fat, he would still have 12 lbs of excess fat on his body. Each pound of fat provides 3,500 calories of accessible energy, so that means he has 42,000 readily available calories to use for energy. The point is - he has plenty of fat stores to fuel his workout even at 8% body fat. When your body is using fat for fuel, you have everything you need.

WILL I LOSE MUSCLE WITHOUT EATING AS MUCH PROTEIN AND CARBS?

There are actually many bodybuilders who eat a ketogenic diet, so don't worry, you can definitely build muscle while eating a moderate amount of protein on a LCHF diet.

SHOULD WE FOLLOW NET CARBS OR TOTAL CARBS?

When you're counting carbs you'll hear people talk about net carbs or total carbs. So, what's the difference? Net carbs are basically total carbs minus fiber. While net carbs would technically be more accurate, the problem is many products don't list soluble and insoluble fiber. There is no legal definition for net carbs; therefore it's not regulated by the FDA on food labels and calculations can vary by each manufacturer.

Insoluble fiber does not dissolve in water and is not absorbed by your body. Insoluble fiber helps with regular bowel movements and moves waste through your body steadily. When your body passes insoluble fiber through without absorbing it, there is no impact on your blood glucose levels, therefore one could subtract this from the carb count.

Soluble fiber creates a viscous solution when introduced to water.

So, if counting net carbs... (if this bores you skip this paragraph)

[Subtract the amount of insoluble fiber from the carbohydrate count.]

If the remaining fiber is more than 5 grams after subtracting the insoluble fiber, subtract half of the soluble fiber.

For example, if there are 8 grams of soluble fiber, reduce the carbohydrate count by 4 grams. Do not subtract any of the soluble fiber if there are less than 5 grams.

Then look at the sugar alcohols. If there are more than 5 grams of sugar alcohols, subtract half that amount from the total carbohydrates. If Erythritol is the only sugar alcohol listed, you may not subtract any sugar alcohols.]

Sound complicated? It is. And many manufacturers do not list soluble vs insoluble because they don't have to. And because it's not regulated, many manufacturers subtract all of the fiber and sugar alcohols to arrive at net carbs, which isn't accurate.

That's why I keep it simple and go by total carbs.

DOES SHAKEOLOGY HAVE A LOT OF CARBS?

Actually, no. Plus, I think counting total carbs for Shakeology is misleading. We do know where the fiber comes from and we do know that it's certified low glycemic (has little effect on your blood sugar). The density of nutrients in it as well as the protein content it contains means you're not going to get a significant rise of blood sugar from Shakeology because it has plenty of protein. Also, the few carbs it has in it are going to help transport the protein to your muscles - especially if you use it post workout. Just the whole makeup of Shakeology and how the foods work together (whole food assimilation) is not going to create an insulin spike - which we know because it's certified low glycemic.

So, you are completely safe and justified to count net carbs in Shakeology. And remember - nobody got fat from drinking Shakeology - whether you're on a LCHF lifestyle or not.

WHAT'S THE DEAL WITH KETONE TEST STRIPS, AND ARE THEY WORTH GETTING?

Ketones will spill into the urine ONLY when there is more in the blood than is being used as fuel by the body at that particular moment. I was testing almost every time I peed for awhile to see how it would differ during the day. Some people say to test first thing in the morning because that's when it's the lowest - so if it's positive then, you know you'll be in ketosis the whole day. I never tested first thing in the morning though.

It doesn't have to be much. Trace to small is fine. It shows there are ketones and that's all that matters. If it's too dark that usually means you're dehydrated, not that you're burning more fat.

The test strips are not the be all end all. Some people never show in ketosis using them. Hopefully, you do, but if you're losing weight and feeling good, then don't worry about it. There are lots of reasons for them to be negative... you may have exercised or worked a few hours previously, so your muscles would have used up the ketones as fuel, thus there will be no excess. You may have had a lot of liquids to drink, so the urine is more diluted. Or the strips are not fresh, or the lid was not on tight and some moisture got in.

Some low carbs dieters NEVER show above trace or negative even, yet they burn fat and lose weight just fine. If you're losing weight, your clothes are getting looser, you're feeling good, and not hungry all the time - then you are successfully in ketosis.

Also, once your body becomes efficient at using ketones for energy it won't produce more than it needs - which means the strips will be negative because excess won't be in the urine, but ketones are present.

So why use them? Because in the beginning being able to SEE if it's positive is awesome. Also, if it's positive then you can also test to see if you get kicked out of ketosis after having carbs... or how quickly you get back into ketosis after having carbs. They can be a motivational tool to help you get back on track knowing that you'll be testing soon to see how you're doing. It's also nice to verify how you're feeling instead of guessing or hoping.

The bottom line - strips only indicate what's happening in the urine at that moment. Ketosis happens in the blood and body tissues. If you're showing even a small amount, then you are in ketosis, and fat-burning is taking place. Don't get hung up on the ketone sticks. If you do want them, you'll find them in the Diabetic Care isle of your local drug store - they say "for Diabetes or Low Carb Dieters".

RECIPES

Chocolate Peanut Butter Fat Bombs (these are great if you're low on fats for the day - and a fun treat!)

18g ghee
18g coconut oil
32g natural peanut butter
1 packet stevia (optional)
Melt, stir, freeze for 30-60 min, enjoy!
Recipe made four ice cubes
Macros for each ice cube:
Calories: 133
Fat: 13g
Carbs: 2g
Protein: 2g

90 Second Bread (this is great if you're craving bread!)

3 TBS almond flour
1 egg
1/2 tsp baking powder
1 1/2 TBS butter

Cook in the microwave for 90 seconds, cut in half. (I like to toast mine)

Keto Lemonade (perfect pick me up, helps with initial side effects during the first week, and a great cocktail alternative when poured over ice!)

    4 cups water
    1/2 packet Energize
    1/4 tsp Himalayan salt
    4 TBS lemon juice or the juice of 1 lemon

FAVORITE PRODUCTS

My non-negotiable products that I use every day have an *

SHAKEOLOGY

Vegan Vanilla and Vegan Chocolate are my favorites; raw micronutrients and protein.

https://teambeachbody.com/shop/-/shopping/MDSUSH311G?referringRepId=1521343

SHAKEOLOGY BOOST

Digestive Health Boost: Add to shake for extra fiber which is important on LCHF diets. I only use 1/3 scoop daily. I used Magnesium for regularity in the beginning, but for long term additional fiber is the way to go, not magnesium.

https://teambeachbody.com/shop/-/shopping/SHKFiberBoost?referringRepId=1521343

BEACHBODY PERFORMANCE LINE

Energize Pre-Workout: One scoop always before my workouts to replenish my body and get the best natural energy, increased performance and focus. Also a 1/4 scoop when I drink Keto lemonade - yum! I do not count this during my fast since I use it as intended (before movement). Your body will burn through it right away.

https://teambeachbody.com/shop/-/shopping/BBPEnergize?referringRepId=1521343

COLLAGEN

Bone Broth Collagen, by Dr. Axe is the one I use; I add one Tbs to my shake - supports joints, muscles, skin, gut, brain health. As we age our bodies naturally produce less collagen, so supplementing is beneficial. http://amzn.to/2sbgrzJ

Premium Collagen Peptides, grass-fed: http://amzn.to/2qRu6bq

Ghee

Fourth and Heart Vanilla Ghee I use this daily in my coffee! http://amzn.to/2rYiml0

Fourth and Heart Pink Salt Grass-Fed Ghee http://amzn.to/2rNwpiK

Fourth and Heart Original Grass-Fed Ghee http://amzn.to/2rFk26j

MCT OIL/COCONUT OIL

Bulletproof Brain Octane Oil is what I use; 2 tsp added to my coffee for the purest C8 MCT - supports metabolism, brain health, and fat burning! http://amzn.to/2rYj08u

Nature's Way MCT Oil http://amzn.to/2rNCGef

Premium MCT Oil http://amzn.to/2sxQkQT

Coconut Oil, Nature's Made http://amzn.to/2sb7Tc5

SWEETENERS

Swerve Confectioners http://amzn.to/2synAHQ

VITAMINS/SUPPLEMENTS

Vitamin D, by Dr. Axe; almost everyone needs more Vitamin D http://amzn.to/2rYuGlf

Magnesium, Nature's Made; will help with initial side effects and regularity as you get started on the plan. http://amzn.to/2rNIPYc

For Fun! (I use these when I don't have Fat Bombs made)

Bliss Nut-Butters (Peanut Butter with Chia Seeds and Saigon Cinnamon) http://amzn.to/2zFAVUJ

Coconut Peanut Butter http://amzn.to/2rNvor6

Lilly's Dark Chocolate Chips (stevia sweetened) http://amzn.to/2sxISFb

Stur Water Enhancer (great to make a low-carb alcoholic beverage) http://amzn.to/2rNCFXX

Further Reading

Fat For Fuel, by Dr. Mercola http://amzn.to/2rYkyil

The Obesity Code, Unlocking The Secrets Of Weightloss
http://amzn.to/2sxS3p8

Sources

Intermittent Fasting: fitness.mercola.com

Hunger Hormones: https://draxe.com/ghrelin/

Carbohydrates and excess fat stores: https://draxe.com/visceral-fat/